Child Psychological Abuse Awareness & Prevention

BY BEN RODGERS

ISBN: 9798323929856

Published in the United States of America

COVER

This book is dedicated to my children and my family. They've been used as weapons to hurt me... brainwashed to the point that they don't know the difference between a good parent and a bad parent. I haven't spoken to my daughter in over 5 years, and I haven't had a relationship with my family in over a decade.

The false accusations against me have given me depression, PTSD, and suicidal thoughts. I genuinely love my kids and family. I miss them every day. My heart is broken, and I'd do anything to get them back in my life.

The purpose of this book is not to trash my ex-wife's reputation. I make it very clear that both men and women can be alienators.

There are 17 alienating strategies, so it's important to see real-life examples of these to understand how it works.

Parental alienation happens every day, it's a combination of interference, isolation, and manipulation. My goal is to help educate people about how child psychological abuse works and why it's a crime.

I hope my story brings awareness to a serious mental illness and provides the tools necessary to prevent long-term and irreversible damage to children.

ABOUT US

CPAAP is the only training program for Attachment System (Disorders) awareness, and Child Psychological Abuse prevention. Our tried-and-true system is based on the research and expertise shared between the leading experts in this field.

We pride ourselves on helping our clients understand family dynamics correctly and are sure that you will leave our sessions more prepared than you have ever been before to protect our children.

TRAINING SESSIONS

Our sessions are meticulously planned by our trainer and are designed in a manner geared toward domestic violence awareness, prevention, and treatment. Your time is valuable, so our goal is to best prepare you while taking up the least amount of your time possible. Training sessions will cover the following subjects:

- My Story
- Development of a Healthy Child
- High-Conflict Divorce
- Attachment System (Disorders)
- How To Diagnose Parental Alienation Correctly
- Symptoms Of Psychological Abuse (Red Flags and Patterns)
- 10 Things Alienated Kids Won't Admit
- Improve Research/Testing/Monitoring
- Treatment Plan
- What Does Parental Alienation Sound Like?
- The Adult Child

BACKGROUND

WHEREAS the Trainer holds significant expertise in Attachment Disorders/PA and offers training services in awareness and prevention for which the Client would like to engage, the Trainer is not a doctor, psychologist, or attorney.

Please contact 911 in case of emergency or get help from a licensed professional.

CONTINUING EDUCATION

Continuing Education (CE) credits are available. Please contact the Trainer for details.

Ben Rodgers can be reached at 512-968-6163 or brodgers2222@gmail.com

REFERENCES

Dr. Amy Baker

Dr. Bill Bernet

Dr. Jennifer Harman

Dr. Craig Childress

Dr. Robert Evans

Children 4 Tomorrow

CHAPTER 1: MY STORY

Any first-year family law student would've been able to help me win custody of my kids and prevent them from being fatherless, IF they were trained in child psychological abuse. The reality is that parents can easily spend $50,000-$100,000 fighting for custody of their children, and still not "win" anything.

I've never physically or sexually harmed anyone, I never cheated on my ex-wife, I'm not a bank robber or a crackhead, I have no psychological or psychiatric disorders, I never missed a child support payment in 10 years, and I genuinely love my children and family. So why has everyone turned against me?

It's a complicated story, like a 1,000-piece jigsaw puzzle with no image on the box to reference. It's also a sad story watching my children and family turn into living zombies with no empathy, no remorse, and no common sense.

About 10 therapists misdiagnosed my case and were complicit with child abuse, 6 judges put a restraining order on me with no evidence of violence, and the police department failed to enforce a (FELONY) Penal Code. False accusations from my family has given me depression, PTSD, and suicidal thoughts.

I've been accused of going postal, terrorizing people, kidnapping, abandoning my children and ruining my family. My father called me a child abuser, he said that I was bat-shit crazy, and that I belong in prison. His only advice to me was to stop "complaining" about my ex-wife. Huh?

From an outsider looking in, my ex-wife appears to be a great mother. She never physically harmed our children, she has a good job and lives in a nice home, she fed our kids well, she bought nice clothes for our kids, she took our kids to all their football and cheerleading events and made sure that our kids got good grades in school.

Why are my children rejecting me???

Why is my family attacking me???

Why are the therapists and judges treating me like a criminal???

I must've done something "wrong" since I don't live in a bubble after all. I'm human, I have feelings and I get upset just like everyone else. What I learned is that the problem has nothing to do with my behavior at all. Let's start from the beginning...

After graduating college, I moved to California and within a few months met my future wife. It was love at first sight; I couldn't get her off my mind. It literally took me five years to get my first date with her. I was broke, had no job and no car, and she wasn't about to get involved with me until I got my act together.

So, I worked hard for five years to establish myself and prove that I was worthy of her love. Then one day, I went into the restaurant where she worked, asked her out on a date and gave her my phone number. We dated for a few years, got married, moved in together and had two children.

Early in the relationship, I found out that my ex-wife was fatherless, and she always said terrible things about him. I didn't think much about it at the time.

Apparently, her father (grandpa) woke up on a Tuesday morning and decided to "abandon" her for the rest of his life. I thought that was very strange but couldn't figure out why he would do that. It wasn't until years later that I figured out what really happened. Grandpa simply fell in love with another woman, so grandma became very jealous and bitter, and ran him off.

Grandma began a campaign of denigration against grandpa. She manipulated my ex-wife who was just an eight-year-old child at the time, to hate grandpa.

Grandma isolated grandpa, and now my ex-wife is isolating me. Grooming and isolation runs in her family. This type of family history is a huge red flag and pattern that most therapists don't take into consideration when assessing their patients.

My ex-wife and I had a rocky relationship for 14 years. Whenever we would argue, she would give me the silent treatment for about 3 days. She never apologized for anything, and constantly devalued me. If she wanted to go left and I wanted to go right, then we would get in a fight. I'd have to give her everything that she wanted to keep the peace. Compromising was not an option; it was her way or the highway. I was married to a narcissist, so having a relationship with her was not possible no matter how hard I tried. By the end of our relationship, I was afraid and outnumbered, so I just gave up. It was safer to keep my mouth shut and not voice my opinion about anything.

She threatened to divorce me for the entire time that we were together.

She threatened to divorce me if I grew a beard. She threatened to divorce me if I got a vasectomy. She threatened to divorce me if I wanted to visit an old friend. She threatened to divorce me if we didn't spend our entire savings account on her education, and then she filed for divorce 45 days after she graduated. It was her plan all along to be debt free, get the house, child support and custody of our children so she could isolate them from me.

I just wanted to get out of the marriage, but she wanted me to suffer for leaving her.

My ex-wife physically assaulted me 3x while we were separating. I filed a police report, but nobody cared. I was afraid of her, so I moved into a gated community, and caught her trespassing shortly thereafter. I complained about that as well, but nobody cared. The court ordered my ex-wife to sign over the title to one of our vehicles.

When I went over to her house to get the papers signed, her stepfather came charging out and started spitting in my face. He stepped on my foot which made it more difficult for me to get away from him. Grandma and my ex-wife were inside the house, and they took the kids into the back bedroom.

They turned up the volume on the TV as loud as it would go to drown out the argument on the front porch, instead of trying to stop the fight. The reason that he attacked me is because he was trying to provoke me into a fight.

I would've gone to jail for hitting him on his property. I filed a police report, but nobody cared. My family told me to stop complaining.

Just a few months after we separated my mother came to visit and stayed at my ex-wife's house for a week. They got drunk together and conspired against me to see if I would give up my designated time with our children. They were "testing" me. My ex-wife would only allow me to see our children 4 days per month (every other weekend), so of course I refused to give up any of my designated time with the kids. They all accused me of being selfish and unreasonable. I complained to my mother that she was being disrespectful and hurtful... but she got mad and accused me of trying to break up their friendship.

At this point, my family was so angry with me for complaining that they threatened to cut me off for the rest of their lives and wanted nothing to do with me. My father insisted that I should love my ex-wife unconditionally. Per his request I sent her two apology letters, and all I heard back was silence.

My ex-wife signed our children up for tutoring on my designated weekends without my permission or consent, which was a violation of our court orders. She wanted to minimize my time with our kids, instead of creating good memories with them. Whenever I tried to contact my ex-wife to discuss school or extracurricular activities for our children, she would contact her attorney and accuse me of harassing her and that she was afraid of me. In turn, her attorney would tell the judges that I was causing problems, so the cards were stacked against me.

My ex-wife will cry and tell our kids that they're abandoning and hurting her by leaving her alone on holidays. So, our children believe that they're betraying their mother by spending holidays with me.

My ex-wife uses our children and my entire family like pawns to hurt me. She rewards our children for cancelling plans with me. She starts crying so our kids will give her what she wants. She gets angry and threatens our kids if they want to spend time with me.

She constantly lies to my family to make them believe that I'm a bad father and a bad person. She uses my family like Flying Monkeys to hurt me and turn them against me. Since my ex-wife refuses to communicate with me directly, she forces our children to be in the middle of our spousal conflicts. To make matters worse, she would schedule multiple activities for our children on my designated time without my permission or consent. All the logistics of dropping off and picking up our kids had to go through my daughter. Not one therapist or judge was concerned about Mom using our kids like puppets or refusing to coparent. My child support was used to help pay for school, food, clothes and other activities... but Mom told our kids "the only thing that child support is used for is to pay for dog food." I complained about this too, but it fell upon deaf ears.

Three years after we separated, my ex-wife lied to everyone and said she "forgot" that our children were supposed to spend Christmas with me. She took them on vacation instead of dropping them off like the divorce orders required.

This was a clear violation of Texas Penal Code 25.03 – Interference With Custody. It's a FELONY and carries up to 2 years prison sentence because it's the same thing as a child abduction. I filed a police report and complained to the judges... but nobody cared. My entire family was also complicit with this criminal behavior, and never held her accountable for anything. My daughter said that she was afraid to ask her mother for additional time with me, because she didn't want to "poke the bear".

If I got stuck in traffic and showed up just a few minutes late to pick up our children, my ex-wife would say that I forfeited my entire weekend and threaten to withhold them.

One weekend I went to pick up the children at my designated time, and my ex-wife started screaming at me saying that they were her kids, not our kids.

She falsely accused me of "abandoning" our kids and said that I was trying to "force" them out of their house. I just walked away and cried on my way home.

The next morning, I had a full-blown panic attack when the realization hit me that I was going to lose my children and family forever. It felt like I was having a heart attack.

My daughter's behavior had substantially changed by this time. When she came to visit me on weekends, she was rude, disrespectful, and constantly talking back to me. If I tried to do my job as a parent and punish her (take her phone away), she would threaten to stop coming over.

She had developed the exact same narcissistic behaviors as her mother... no empathy, no remorse and lack of ambivalence. My son was afraid to voice his opinion, so he stayed quiet most of the time.

A little while later the family court judge put a restraining order on me and gave me a no contact order. I was not allowed to say Happy Birthday or Merry Christmas to my children for 3 years. The judge also ordered me to get a psychological evaluation. Ironically, the therapist reported that my ex-wife was interfering in my relationship with the children.

I tried to explain this to my family, but they refused to listen and accused me of not doing enough to help my ex-wife. They all believe that my ex-wife is the Target Parent because I complain about her. Their assessment is wrong. Little do they realize that children reject the target parent and favor the alienating parent. I volunteered to attend anger management therapy. That turned out to be a complete waste of time since the therapist told me to "go home" after only 2 meetings. The therapist advised me to choose my words more carefully, and offered no explanation as to why my custody was revoked. My ex-wife got remarried and her new husband was doing everything he could to replace me. He would show up to all my kids' football and cheerleading games and pick fights with me. Two of his children moved in with him, and they both moved out shortly afterwards because of my ex-wife's behavior.

The judge ordered me to go to reunification therapy with my children. The therapist made me write an apology letter for my bad behavior since I was still complaining about my ex-wife. I asked the therapist if she had ever heard of parental alienation, and she threw her arms up in the air like she scored a touchdown and said, "I know everything there is to know about parental alienation!" The therapist never acknowledged that my ex-wife assaulted me, was isolating the children or committed felony interference. She refused to allow me to see my children. So, I fired her.

At some point my daughter asked if she could move in with me. My ex-wife got extremely angry and threatened her with the ultimatum "if you move in with your dad, I'll never speak to you again as long as I live!"

Same story with the next 9 therapists... no contact with my children, no acknowledgement of my ex-wife's behavior, and all of them demanding that I get rid of my evidence and stop complaining. One therapist told me to "take unequivocal responsibility for my behavior."

In short, the therapists believe that it's worse for me to complain about my ex-wife, than it is to hold her accountable for assault, isolating our kids and criminal behavior.

Multiple therapists misdiagnosed me of being "stuck in my lane" because I was focused on my ex-wife. I simply want to have a peaceful and enjoyable relationship with my kids without having to worry about my ex-wife interfering in our relationship. Two different judges gave my ex-wife a gag order and told her to stop speaking to my family about me. That was violated on a regular basis.

Over the years my family has been so poisoned by my ex-wife that they actually believe I'm:

-Not picking the kids up on time

-Not doing what I'm supposed to

-Doing things that are unwanted and unwelcome

-Owe my ex-wife money

None of these accusations are true... it's all frivolous nonsense. My family lives 2,000 miles away and gets all of their information from my ex-wife. My family doesn't realize that they're being USED like a weapon to hurt me. They're afraid of the truth, so they refuse to admit that they've been brainwashed.

Of course, I complained about these false accusations and tried to defend myself, but that just led to more fighting. It took me a long time to figure out that my ex-wife started bad-mouthing me long before we got divorced. At our final court hearing, my ex-wife pressed charges and tried to throw me in prison for 4 years because I violated the restraining order. All

I did was text my son about rescheduling a counseling meeting. I was truly scared for my life at this point. I couldn't afford a lawyer, so I had to defend myself.

Luckily, the judge dismissed the charges. The judge ordered me to pay almost $20,000 for all my ex-wife's legal fees within 60 days and forced me to get another psychological evaluation. Unable to afford that, I was forced to declare bankruptcy.

None of the 10 therapists I went to for help bothered to look at my psychological evaluations. It was a complete waste of time and money. They all have a duty to report child psychological abuse, yet they refused to report anything.

The therapists and judges don't care if they're wrong because they have immunity from their licensing boards. They all accused me of being the alienating parent because I was complaining about my ex-wife. They have everything backwards!

On a more positive note, a few months after the final hearing I got my son back the day he turned 18. I simply called him up and asked if he wanted to go out to dinner for his birthday. My ex-wife could no longer use the corrupt family court system to isolate him. For one year we had a great time fishing, golfing, watching basketball games and going out to dinner every week. My son said that he loved me many times. We had a lot of fun, but he was hurting me at the same time. He refused to spend holidays with me, he forgot my birthday, and he demanded that we avoid talking about his mother.

Then it all came crashing down on Father's Day. My son wanted to go out to dinner with me and told me to make reservations after he got off work. His mother found out about it and got so ANGRY at him that he cancelled our plans. He was afraid of dealing with his mother's aggression and didn't know how to handle the situation. I got very upset and complained about it, so my son blocked me. I haven't talked to him since then. He showed no empathy, no remorse and didn't do anything to repair our relationship.

The year prior my ex-wife took our children out of the country on Father's Day weekend. She planned to hurt me for 6 months while she made plans with them. My family was totally complicit with my ex-wife hurting me on Father's Day because they all knew about the trip. This pattern of my ex-wife isolating our kids on Father's Day is evidence of an Attachment System (Disorder).

Most recently, my father called me right before my daughter's college graduation. He was screaming, threatening, and demanding that I stay at home instead of attending the graduation. He said that if I go to the graduation, he'd never speak to me again as long as he lives. I went to the graduation anyway and enjoyed watching her special day. I'm very proud of her!

My ex-wife believes that she's entitled to Father's Day and Mother's Day. She gets angry and threatens our children for trying to have a relationship with me. She is USING our children to hurt me. She has no reference of shared parenting since she grew up fatherless. She believes that I'm trying to harm her and our children, which means that she's suffering from persecutory delusions. Nobody has ever held her responsible for physical violence, isolating our children or criminal behavior. To be clear, any parent who unjustly isolates a child from the other parent, is a child abuser. Children need both parents.

The purpose of my story is to let people know the real reason that my children are rejecting me. They're afraid of their mother's wrath and being CUT-OFF by her. She'll get angry and punish our children for trying to have a relationship with me... she treats them like her property and can't detach from them.

It's important to understand that my ex-wife is suffering from an Attachment System (Disorder). She doesn't know how to process sharing our children or the value of our children having a Dad.

Parental alienation is counter-intuitive because our children give their mother reflexive support and never say a bad word about her. Our kids constantly denigrate me to appease her. She is forcing our children to either be motherless or fatherless, they must choose only one parent. Induced compliance is psychological abuse... it's Domestic Violence. I genuinely hope that my children figure out what's happening to them and have the courage to stand up for themselves.

I also hope that my ex-wife gets counseling to resolve her own issues. Lastly, I hope my family realizes that they're punishing the wrong person, and I get to speak to them again someday. My heart has been broken into a million pieces, and I just want the pain to end.

CHAPTER 2: DEVELOPMENT OF A HEALTHY CHILD

In a perfect world, absent of any physical or sexual abuse, a child will develop a unique and complex bond with both parents.

The mother-child bond is vastly different than the father-child bond, yet both are equally important for the child's emotional and psychological development.

Parents should recognize the value that they each contribute and encourage the child to bond with the other parent.

After divorce there is increased pressure for a child to learn how to navigate conflicts, settle disagreements, and restore relationships. Our family court system is incentivized to separate families which creates a tremendous amount of stress on the natural parent-child bonding.

Unstable parents can take advantage of this system and use the child as a weapon to harm the other parent.

This toxic combination of legal and mental wrangling is confusing for a child and should be dealt with in therapy, not litigation.

If a parent is physically or sexually abusing a child, then law enforcement should arrest that harmful parent immediately.

If a parent is isolating, manipulating, and threatening a child, then therapists and judges should remove the child from that parent.

When a child can successfully avoid conflicts, set boundaries, de-escalate issues and repair relationships... it shows that the child has developed healthy emotional and psychological behaviors.

CHAPTER 3: HIGH-CONFLICT DIVORCE

Research shows that 50/50 shared parenting is best for children. For the most part, problems are minimal for separated families when there's evidence of coparenting, mutual respect and obeying the divorce orders. It's normal for children to be emotionally hurt when parents get divorced because they're dealing with the death of a family.

In low-conflict divorces, the trauma and sadness can typically be dealt with by counseling, a good support group, and time to adjust to the new reality.

Attachment System (Disorders) aka "Parental Alienation" is typically seen in high conflict divorces.

It involves the deliberate and malicious actions by one parent to use the child as a pawn to hurt the other parent. It happens slowly, methodically, and covertly.

Most therapists, judges, attorneys, law enforcement, schools and child protective services are not trained or qualified to understand the family dynamics correctly.

Federal law Title IV-D creates the perfect opportunity for the custodial parent to control, brainwash and weaponize the child.

Using lawyers and judges who know little about the family to decide who is the "best parent" is extremely destructive.

This type of toxic custody battle forces the child to be caught in the middle of the spousal conflict and encourages the child to choose sides.

Standard visitation is harmful to families:

*Family courts, attorneys and therapists profit from separating families.

*Child Support can cause one parent to be broke and very stressed out. (Fines, prison, garnished wages, suspended driver's license, etc.)

*Law enforcement and CPS don't handle psychological abuse.

*Texas Penal Code 25.03 - Interference With Custody (it's a FELONY)

-Police, Judges and Attorney General refuse to enforce it!

There are mild to severe levels of Attachment System (Disorders)/Parental Alienation and special training is necessary to diagnose it properly.

CHAPTER 4: ATTACHMENT SYSTEM (DISORDERS)

Children do NOT reject their parents. The bond between a child and their parents is a deep motivational system of the brain and is almost unbreakable.

Evaluating why a child would reject a loving parent is complicated and frequently misunderstood since it's like Stockholm Syndrome. Most people get everything backwards!

Most therapists are not trained in Attachment System (Disorders)/Parental Alienation, so they're operating outside their area of expertise and scope of competence by offering "reunification therapy."

Let's start by learning some important pathologies and concepts...

Narcissistic Personality Disorder

-Characterized by inflated self-worth, and devaluing others

Borderline Personality Disorder

-Characterized by an unstable and distorted sense of self

Pathogenic Enmeshment

-A parent's unhealthy attachment to the child

Persecutory Delusions

-One parent's beliefs that the other parent is trying to harm the child

Induced Compliance

-Manipulating and forcing a child to contradict their own beliefs

False Accusations

-Allegations of wrongdoing that are untrue

Cross-Generational Coalition

-Triangulation between a parent and child against the other parent

All these abusive behaviors may be displayed simultaneously by the narcissistic parent to hurt the other parent. However, just like a cult, fear and brainwashing are well hidden. Anyone who studies Attachment System (Disorders) must realize that the family dynamics are counter intuitive. The child is held hostage, effectively coerced, and seduced into acting like a spy for the narcissistic parent. Then, the narcissistic parent validates those bad behaviors by rewarding the child with praise and attention.

Alienating parents will blatantly lie to everyone and say that they want the child to have a relation-ship with the other parent.

Parental Alienation is a criminal issue... NOT a civil/custody issue.

Everyone should be aware of:

-Domestic violence
-Intent to hurt
-Criminal behavior
-Hostage taking
-Coercive control
-Enmeshment

CHAPTER 5: HOW TO DIAGNOSE PARENTAL ALIENATION

Parental Alienation is a made-up term and isn't recognized by the American Psychological Association, DSM-5, schools, or the family court system. Judges will try to reconnect a parent and child by ordering "reunification therapy," but this is a made-up term as well. Diagnosing child psychological abuse correctly means using well-established psychological constructs, not theories and made-up terms.

For clarification purposes, here are two (made-up) terms that are critical to understand since most people get them wrong...

Alienating Parent
-The parent who is favored by the child
-The parent who is using the child to hurt the other parent
-The parent who interferes with the child and other parent
-The parent who isolates the child from the other parent
-The parent who makes false accusations about the other parent

-The parent who typically has <u>primary custody</u> of the child

Target Parent
-The parent who is being rejected by the child
-Typically "complaining" about the other parent
-Typically comes across as "angry" and "stuck in their lane"
-Typically the <u>non-custodial</u> parent

The easiest and best way to determine which parent is the alienator is by using Dr. Amy Baker's 4-part model:

1. Did the child and rejected parent have a loving relationship PRIOR to divorce?

2. Absence of physical or sexual abuse by rejected parent

3. Alienating Parent Strategies

*Poisonous messages to child that the other parent is unloving, unsafe, and unavailable

*Limiting contact and communication

*Erasing and replacing the targeted parent

*Encouraging child to betray the target parent

*Undermining the authority of the target parent

4. Symptoms of child psychological abuse

*Lack of empathy
*Lack of remorse
*Lack of ambivalence
*Frivolous reasons for rejecting the target parent
*Reflexive support for alienating parent

When someone sees these behaviors in a child... they need to understand that the child is living in FEAR of the alienating parent, and the child is being FORCED to choose only one parent.

The child is AFRAID to stand up for themself because setting boundaries with the alienator is typically met with aggression, punishment, threats, and ultimatums. Most people don't understand that the child favors the parent who's threatening and isolating the child from the other parent.

Another strategy is that the alienator will undermine visitation rights by suggesting tempting alternatives, and then rewarding the child for cancelling plans with the target parent. An alienator may also make the child feel guilty for spending time with the target parent. For instance, Mom may say to the child "please don't abandon me on Christmas, you're hurting me by spending Christmas with your Dad." Often, the alienator will PROVOKE a fight by scheduling activities for the child on the target parent's designated time, without consent.

Alienators are master manipulators!

Therapists need to be trained in coercive control, grooming, social isolation, gaslighting, red flags and pattern recognition. Alienators fail to recognize their own behavior.

The family operates like a cult... the narcissistic alienator seems charismatic and loving but controls the child behind closed doors by threatening and punishing the child. Therapists should separate the alienator and child, then monitor the alienator for compliance.

When alienators are exposed or held accountable, they'll decompensate and ostracize. Some alienators will murder their own child just to prevent the target parent from having a relationship with the child.

Reunification therapy is criticized by many because it means removing the child from the alienating parent and placing the child with the target parent for 90 days.

Outsiders don't understand why a therapist would force a child to be with a rejected parent. In rare instances, both parents can be alienators.

CHAPTER 6: SYMPTOMS OF CHILD PSYCHOLOGICAL ABUSE

Lack of Empathy

Lack of Remorse

Lack of Ambivalence

Frivolous reasons for rejecting the target parent

Reflexive support for alienating parent

Child is living in FEAR of being CUT OFF by alienating parent

Child is FORCED to choose only one parent

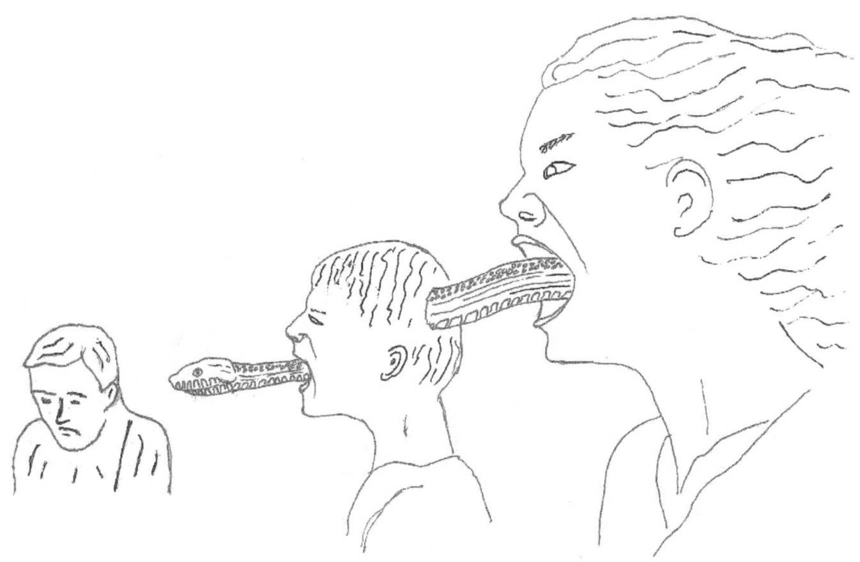

Therapists, judges, law enforcement, CPS, schools, and families should spend less time listening to the parents bad-mouthing each other... and more time listening to the child. Children do NOT reject loving parents!

A child isn't going to set boundaries or tattle-tale on an alienating parent because they're afraid of the consequences. Nor will a child admit that they lack empathy or remorse for the target parent. But the child will give frivolous reasons for rejecting the target parent. After a few years of being told that the target parent is unloving, unsafe, and unavailable the child will actually believe it.

Careful questioning and a tactful approach are necessary to expose where the abuse is coming from. Therapists need to look for the red flags and patterns, without pointing fingers at anyone.

Treatment is more effective when the child is a minor, where a judge can change custody and order an alienating parent to cooperate. Once the child has aged-out of the system, it becomes much more difficult to stop the abuse.

CHAPTER 7: 10 THINGS ALIENATED KIDS WON'T ADMIT

1) Alienator loves to bad-mouth the Target parent

*Kids don't know any different, it's normal to them

*Kids don't know that it's wrong, no comparison

2) Kids don't want to admit that their decisions have been influenced to hate the Target parent. Known as the "independent thinker" phenomenon.

3) Kids want the Target parent to love them

*Brainwashed to think that they were abandoned

*Kids miss the Target parent... inner void that needs to be filled

4) Kids wish things were different with the Target parent

5) Kids say negative things about the Target parent like "selfish, unstable, abandoned", etc.

6) Kids fear getting hurt again

7) Kids feel guilty for spending time with the Target parent

*Betraying the Alienator

8) Kids are hurting inside, but angry outside (mask)

9) Kids can't be themselves, they put up a wall and are guarded

10) Getting close to the Target parent will upset the Alienator

*Kids will be interrogated and CUT OFF by the Alienator

The child can't spend time with, speak about, communicate with, or show love towards a parent they love.

Instead, they must take on the alienator's thoughts and feelings as if they are their own.

A "normal range" parent should be willing to share the child with the other parent, without getting upset.

CHAPTER 8:
RESEARCH/TESTING/MONITORING

Read books by experts (Foundations by Dr. Childress)

Watch videos (YouTube: Parental Alienation - In the Eyes of the Experts)

Join professional PA groups (PASG)

Alienating parents don't want to be exposed, so they won't participate in family counseling.

WARNING: Removing child from alienating parent may result in Domestic Violence

Therapists have a DUTY to report abuse. Protect the child and target parent

-Standards & Ethics 2.01, 2.04 and 9.01

-DSM 5 (V995.51)

CHAPTER 9: TREATMENT PLAN

Parenting Practices Rating Scale (1-4)

*Levels 1 and 2 are deviant-abusive
*Levels 3 and 4 are normal range

3 Strikes You're Out!

*Holds both parents accountable

*Punishment for interfering/isolating the child

The purpose of these tools is to allow the target parent an opportunity to restore the relationship with the child, by removing the alienating parent.

Using a standardized test like the Parenting Practices Rating Scale provides a baseline for therapists to determine which parent may be problematic. Then the family courts need to hold both parents accountable by using the 3 Strikes You're Out! model.

CHAPTER 10: WHAT DOES PARENTAL ALIENATION SOUND LIKE?

1) Dad: Simply picking up the child from Mom's home...

Mom says to the child: "Call me if you need anything!"

*Analysis: Alienating parent (Mom) is displaying narcissistic behaviors by trying to establish superiority over the target parent (Dad). The alienator wants the child to think that the target parent is inadequate. The truth is that Dad and the child don't want or need anything from the alienator.

*Treatment: A good parent would simply tell the child "hope y'all have a nice weekend!"

2) Mom says to child: "You know how I keep telling you that your dad is a bad guy, and he doesn't deserve us. Well today in court the judge agreed with me and now Daddy isn't allowed to see you.

Hopefully one day he will start putting our needs first and he will start being nice to us. I hope he cares enough about you to work on himself."

*Analysis: Mom is making false accusations and displaying Persecutory Delusions. Mom believes that Dad is trying to harm her and the child.

The truth is that Dad is a good guy, never harmed anyone and just wants to see the child. The judge doesn't realize that he/she is being manipulated by the alienator and is complicit with child abuse by putting a restraining order on Dad.

3) Mom says to Dad: "Oops, I forgot that the kids were supposed to spend Christmas with you."

*Analysis: Mom is lying and suffers from an Attachment System (Disorder), she doesn't want Dad to have a relationship with the children.

*Mom committed FELONY child abuse - Interference With Custody

Psychological abuse works both ways, dads can be alienators too!

4) Mom says: I'll pick up the kids on Friday at 6:00 pm

Dad says: "You can discuss that with the kids"

*Analysis: Allowing children to choose their own schedule is a known form of parental alienation.

5) Mom says: I have to work this weekend to pay child support

Dad says to child: "Mom abandoned you"

*Analysis: Alienators twist what happened and turn it into something terrible or offensive. Next, they use this terrible/offensive event as fuel to turn the child against the Target parent.

6) Mom says: "I just want to spend more time with our child"

Dad says: Mom's trying to "force" my child out of the house

*Analysis: Dad clearly has control issues by saying "my" child.

*Dad is suffering from a Persecutory Delusion since he believes that Mom is trying to harm him and the child.

7) Dad says to Child: If you move in with your mom, I'll never speak to you again!

*Analysis: This is an example of induced compliance to isolate the child from Mom.

8) Dad says to Mom: If you don't pay child support, you'll never see your child again!

*Analysis: This is an example of triangulation, by using the child to deal with spousal conflict.

CHAPTER 11: THE ADULT CHILD

When an alienated child grows up, the "fingerprints" of the alienator will be seen on the child. In other words, the adult child will typically have the same narcissistic personality disorder/borderline personality disorder that the alienating parent had. The adult child may feel compelled to get divorced and then isolate their child from the other parent.

Parental alienation can pass from generation to generation. A child that grows up with only one parent will think that it's normal because they have nothing to compare it to. Therefore, the adult alienated child will strive to be a single parent and raise their child the same way. Child abuse "runs in the family."

Attachment System (Disorders)/Parental Alienation ranges from mild to severe... but the damage to a child that's forced to choose only one parent is permanent and irreversible. Parents need to use great care when raising a child and put their "bitter" feelings for the other parent aside. A parent will never be a Superhero if it comes at the expense of the other parent. Parents should always do what's best for the child.

SUMMARY

Unfortunately, around 22 million people are going through what's commonly known as "Parental Alienation" so anyone reading this book should realize that it can happen to them as well.

Our family court system is corrupt, plus most mental health clinicians are uneducated and incompetent when it comes to the dynamics of Attachment System (Disorders).

Parental Alienation is a crime and there's no professional help available. This type of psychological abuse is slow, systematic, and unrecognizable by most people.

My goal is to educate everyone about child psychological abuse because it's easy to prevent with the right training. No child should be forced to choose only one parent... treatment is available.

www.ingramcontent.com/pod-product-compliance
Lightning Source LLC
Chambersburg PA
CBHW051711250726
48653CB00007B/2979